THE
6-FIGURE SALONPRENEUR™

8 Easy Steps to Making $100K Working 3 Days a Week or Less

Alex B. Jones

Thank you Amy! Much success to you! Be great! Alex B.J.

Copyright © 2016 Alex B. Jones. All rights reserved.

No portion of this book may be reproduced mechanically, electronically, or by any other means, including photocopying, without written permission of the publisher. It is illegal to copy this book, post it to a website, or distribute it by any other means without written permission from the publisher.

Alex B. Jones

Alex@AlexBJones.com

Rock Hill, SC

Limits of Liability and Disclaimer of Warranty

The author and publisher shall not be liable for your misuse of this material. This book is strictly for informational and educational purposes.

Warning- Disclaimer

The purpose of this book is to inform and educate. The author and/or publisher do not guarantee that anyone following these techniques, suggestions, tips, tools, or strategies will become successful. The author and/or publisher shall have neither liability nor responsibility to anyone with respect to any loss or damage caused, or alleged to be caused, directly or indirectly, by the information contained in this book.

This dedicated to my best friend, the love of my life and my wonderful wife, Alease.

TABLE OF CONTENT

Introduction	1
Step 1 Create a "6-Figure Mindset"	13
Step 2 "6-Figure Math" & Setting Your Targets	27
Step 3 What's Your Story	41
Step 4 Maximizing Client Value	49
Step 5 Increasing Your FOV's	57
Step 6 Building Your Clientele	61
Step 7 Adjusting Your Prices	71
Step 8 Tracking Your Progress	79
About the Author	85
Additional Products and Services	87
The 6-Figure Salonpreneur™ Progress Tracking Worksheets	88

INTRODUCTION

You are *very* lucky! Not only because you decided to get this book, but because you are a part of an amazing industry, the Beauty Industry. The Beauty Industry gives you tremendous opportunities to express your passion, your creativity, generate unlimited income and create real freedom in your life.

Yet, in an Industry where you are limited only by your imagination and can make as much as you want, the average beauty professional struggles just to make it day by day.

Here are some interesting facts for you...

- there are over 656,400 hairstylists in the U.S.
- the median income is $23,170 per year, $11.40/hour
- 80% of *all* hairstylists make less than $43,350
- the average salon owner gets to keep just 7 cents of every dollar if they have any profit at all
- the typical hairstylist leaves the Industry within 5 years
- most cosmetologists don't know how to market their business
- most hairstylists can barely afford health care premiums
- and is frustrated at their inability to achieve the level of success they really want.

As Founder of The Salonpreneur™ Academy and salon business coach, I see firsthand the struggles, stress, and financial hardships many hairstylists and salon owners experience all across the country.

Sadly, it's not because they aren't nice people. It's not because their hearts aren't in the right place or that they aren't good at what they do. It's because they were never taught what they really need to know to be successful as a salon business owner. They were taught, *"just be good at your craft, work hard, and you'll be successful."* Sadly, this simply is not true. Being a great stylist is only part of the equation for a successful salon business. The other part? Well, just keep reading.

Purpose for This Book

My purpose for writing this book is to provide you, the hairstylist, booth renter, salon suite owner, small business owner and independent beauty professional the essential information you need to transform your salon business, create unlimited income and have the freedom to live on your own terms. When I say independent beauty professional, I'm referring to anyone who provides beauty, health and wellness services and/or products i.e.

hairstylists, makeup artists, nail technicians, brow and lash specialists, massage therapists, estheticians, etc.

This book was created for you to have as a guide and to keep with you until you become a 6-figure earner. The eight steps I lay out are in very simple and easy to understand language that are guaranteed to get you started today on becoming a 6-figure earner and top stylist working 3 days or less a week so you can truly have the freedom to enjoy the life you deserve. But, you must apply them.

In this book, you will...

- Gain amazing clarity and laser focus on your purpose and business strategy
- Know exactly what to say to attract your perfect clients
- how to work 3 days a week or less in your salon
- discover a simple 8-step system to generate at least $100k in revenue
- how to recommend additional services and products without feeling sleazy or pushy
- how to become a top-earner in the beauty industry
- learn how to price your services for maximum profit
- have more confidence and less stress
- and have more time to enjoy life.

Who am I

I am a 22-year Beauty Industry veteran, marketing expert and salon business coach specializing in helping independent hairstylists, booth renters and salon suite owners create successful businesses. I have had the pleasure of owning and operating 3 salons, working as a platform artist and earning a 6-figure income in just 2 ½ short years into my beauty career. I had no prior hairstyling experience or talent. Prior to working in the Beauty Industry, I worked with Kodak Company in Corporate Audit and Marketing and Product Development.

I started with no hairstyling ability and I was able to build a substantial clientele working with my ideal clients who greatly appreciated my services earning well into six-figures. If I can do it, so can you! I have helped hundreds of other hairstylists reach their dreams and I want to show you how to generate the income and freedom you deserve.

Now, I have the pleasure of working 3 days a week, earning a 6-figure income, traveling, enjoying time with my family, and doing what I love…helping other hairstylists, salon and salon suite owners do the same in their business. If I can be successful in the beauty industry, surely you can too!

Why You Must Earn 6 Figures

Reading the title of this book, your co-workers, your friends, family members, or may be even you might be tempted to think, *"I don't need all that", 6-figures ain't necessary* or *"I have a passion for what I do, I don't need to make 6 figures to be happy."* I agree. Money can't buy happiness. But let me assure you, you absolutely should and must earn a minimum of 6-figures to live relatively comfortable and to give yourself and your family some amount of security and options in life. I'm not saying you can't be happy making less. I am saying that stress, worry and discontent of not having enough money to take care of life's necessities, spend time with your kids, handle emergencies, give your family more options in life can and does stress you reducing the likelihood of you being happy.

Will constantly being told "NO" you can't do the things you want in life by the amount of money you have make you happier? Will *not* having enough time and flexibility to do the things you most enjoy doing because your money situation, or lack of it, says "no, you gotta get back to work?!" Having money doesn't mean you will be happy. But *not* having financial freedom certainly won't either! Anyone who said money can't buy happiness is right. But, they're also probably *broke and wish they had more money.*

I've been there too! I know very well what it feels likes to not have money. To have the desire to do things but my pockets tell me "NO". I know the sinking feeling of wanting to do things for my family and not be able to. Or even not be able to take care of the basic necessities of life, food, shelter or my health because I didn't have enough to cover it all. Just having enough is *not* enough.

Here's a very simplified example of why you need to earn more:

6-figure stylist	$100,000
Average weekly booth or salon suite rent	$250/week
Weeks per year	52 weeks
Yearly salon rent total	-$13,000
Yearly product expenses	-$5,000
Other miscellaneous expenses	-$5,000
Income after expenses	$77,000
Minimum Taxes (20%) on $77K	-$15,400
Money left for you and your family	$61,600
Average cost of living for a family of 2 in the U.S……..	$46,246*
family of 4 in the U.S…………….	$64,741*

*According to Economic Policy Institute's Family Budget Calculator. http://www.epi.org/resources/budget/

And these cost of living figures are just the basics. They do not take into account any savings, retirement, or children college tuition. The numbers also do not factor in when you, the self-employed hairstylists and salon owners ***are not*** working, are on vacation, or can't work due to illness or some other unforeseen situation, your income completely stops. You are forced to do whatever is necessary to come in to work come hell or high water, sick or hurt. With 80% of all beauty professionals making less than $43,000, most are already behind in terms of their income.

There is obviously a disconnect between we can *potentially* make in the Beauty Industry and how much we *actually* make. You can see why so many are frustrated, struggling and chose to leave the Industry. But, in an Industry where we are able to make as much as we want, how can it be that we continue to struggle? To avoid this outcome for yourself, becoming a 6-figure earner must become your #1 priority.

Why 3 Days a Week?

Over time, we have become so conditioned to spend most of our life earning *a living* and very little time *having a life*. Those are two very different things. We get up every day, spending the best and majority of our day working. Working to pay bills. Working to have money to live. Working to survive! Where did we get the idea that this is what life is all about? Is this really what you were created to do?

Now, you may choose to work more than 3 days a week. And that's okay. But, let it be your decision to work longer rather than doing it because you have to. You and I have but one life to live.

Wouldn't you prefer to work part-time and live full-time? Well, wouldn't you?

Imagine having a clientele full of clients you love working with. Envision yourself earning more than you ever thought possible, spending lots of time with your family, going on vacations, living stress-free with the security that comes from having abundant finances. If you use this powerful yet simple 8-step strategy I'm going to share, you will go from wherever you are now in your salon business to generating a 6-figure income *and* have the freedom to enjoy it.

How to Use this Book

This book is designed for you to keep it with you on your journey to 6-figures and freedom. Here's how to use it for maximum benefit

1. Start at the beginning and read completely through the book. Get familiar with the concepts.
2. Set aside 1 hour at the beginning of the week, preferably on a Sunday and work through it.
3. Start at the beginning and in order. Each step builds on the other, so complete them in order.
4. Set aside 15 minutes in the morning before starting your day and 30 minutes at night preparing for the next day.

5. Be sure to track your progress and stick to your schedule
6. Talk with your accountability partner once a week.

Weekly Activities

Take time at the beginning of your week to review the past week. This will give you some perspective on what's going well and not so well. You can determine your biggest areas for improvement. This puts you in position to plane your week ahead. Review and planning are cornerstones to success and earning 6-figures in your business. Passing over these activities will put your effort at a significant disadvantage. Give yourself the time it takes to win.

Daily Activities

Take time daily to do your affirmations and follow your daily plan. Execute the plan you lay out. "Eat the frog" which means if you got to do something that's difficult, unpleasant or challenging, do it first. Write down your results and prepare your daily activities for the next day. Don't fit your life into a small budget. Expand your vision and income to afford the life you want.

I encourage you to get several copies of this book and share them with your colleagues and co-workers so you can go this journey together and hold each other accountable. Also as your goals changes you'll want to have a new book for your new goals, contact list, daily activities, and tracker sheet. Remember, this is designed to help you create wealth in your life. This is NOT the time to be cheap. Cheap thinking leads to cheap results. Invest yourself, your business and those around you!

At The Salonpreneur™ Academy, we are always developing new, and exciting ways create the salon business of your dreams. If you would like to get faster results in your salon business, consider joining The Salonpreneur™ SuccessLab Monthly Membership Group. Go to www.alexbjones.com/6figurebookresources for more information on any membership, service or product to help you elevate your success.

Let's begin!

STEP 1
CREATE A
"6-FIGURE MINDSET"

Creating a "6-FIGURE" income in your salon business and wealth in your life begins with establishing a "6-figure" mindset. Everything you see, beautiful buildings, cars, works of art began in someone's mind. Mental thoughts produce physical realities. Creating high income, wealth and success is no different.

A "6-figure" mindset is nothing more than a positive, intentional, and assertive set of thoughts and beliefs about money, your efforts and ability to achieve a 6-figure income. If you aren't generating the income you want, it's likely because you have adapted "lack" or "poor" money thoughts, beliefs or habits. Your thoughts produce lack in reality. I know that sounds harsh, like I'm blaming you. Well, to be honest, I am.

Why?

This can be a hard concept to wrap our brains around, but the sooner you do, the faster you will earn the income you want. If you believe that your financial position in life just happened, was forced on you or that you had no part in creating it, means that other people and outside influences beyond your control determine your income. If you believe that to be true, then it leaves you *powerless* to change your situation and future because you have no power over other people and circumstances. You will be a victim having to accept whatever life and other people throw your way. But the awesome thing is, if you accept full responsibility for your economic circumstances, decisions and future, then you are perfectly positioned to start earning the income you want, seeing the world and doing the things you want for yourself and your family.

Whatever you think and feel about money will manifest itself in your pockets. If you don't believe there is more for you, that is too hard or that you are not deserving of more, then you will never have an abundance of money or wealth. You must change your money beliefs. People without wealth often subconsciously think negative about money and people who possess it. They think things like…

- Rich people are greedy,
- Rich people take from other people,
- I have to work twice as hard to make 2x as much,
- It's hard to get wealthy,
- I'd rather happy than working all the time to make money,
- Money doesn't grow on trees,

- She's filthy rich,
- Rich people are crooks, stingy, or mean,
- I can't win for losing,
- Life is tough,
- Money won't make you happy,
- I'm not lucky enough to win the lottery.

All of the above statements have a lack, negative, poor or limiting belief to them. Money is not attracted to a person with this attitude.

So, how do we change our thinking? How do we develop a "6-figure" mindset? We've already talked about the importance of taking full responsibility for our financial position, decisions and future. Here are some other activities for creating your "6-figure" mindset and mental money magnet.

Your Money Beliefs

List your honest beliefs about money, rich and wealthy people.

- I'll never have enough
- Rich people are assholes
- I can't make enough

- money is happiness
- I want to win lotto
- I need to believe money comes to me easily + unexpectly
- I'm not good enough
-
-
-
-

Are these money beliefs more negative than positive?

more neg than pos

Where did these ideas come from?

growing up?

Thinking and speaking positively is critical to generating more income and achieving wealth. Let's develop more positive beliefs about money and wealth that so you can remind yourself of everyday. For example:

>Rich people are generous and givers
>Rich people put their efforts in areas that produce and deliver greater value
>Money is abundant and flows easily to me
>Rich people think big and take action

- rich people are doers
- rich people help others
- money comes to me in abundance easily & unexpectedly
- I DESERVE to be wealthy
-

- <u>I can save money</u>
- <u>I will retire comfortably</u>

Create Different Habits and Routines

Anything you do consistently, good or bad, becomes a routine or habit. As we said earlier, if you are not where you want to be financially, it's because of what you have done consistently and repeatedly. Success is simply doing the right things, the right way, at the right time, consistently….simple right?! Along with the thinking, people and inputs, you must create routines and habits that support your intentions of generating more income.

Here are a few questions to ask yourself…

Do you buy or spend money to cover up something you don't like about yourself?
<u>yes</u>

Do you buy things to make yourself feel better?
<u>yes</u>

Are you seeking approval or attention from people?
<u>probably yes</u>

Are there things you don't because you don't want to "show" up other people?

Sometimes

Do you have money habits that keep you from have achieving more income and building more wealth?

yes

If so, it's time to create some new habits!

One of the most effective ways to develop a habit of speaking and thinking affirmations. Create your own positive affirmations and repeat them morning, noon and before bed.

Daily Affirmations

I am becoming wealthier and my income is increasing everyday

- I am worth wealth
-
-
-
-

-
-
-
-
-
-
-
-
-

Keep Your Mind On Your Money and Money On Your Mind

"Where attention goes will grow."

Pay attention to how much money you have, how you use it. If you want to generate income and accumulate wealth you must focus your attention on money and wealth. This is what is called being a good steward over your finances. If you are a good steward of little, then you can be trust with more. Otherwise, a fool and his money shall soon part.

Don't do a budget, create a spending plan. Budgets sound and feel too restrictive. That's why nobody likes them let alone stay on them very long. Creating a spending plan, however, gives you the opportunity to develop the list of things you want to have. A spending plan allows you to look at the things you want and develop a great strategy to get them. Determine your list of priorities and then spend according to what is important to your priorities.

Maximize revenue opportunities and create multiple streams. Always be aware of how and where you spend your money. Don't let fear (irrational beliefs) of any kind keep you from taking action: fear of failure, fear of rejection, fear of loss, or even fear of success. The moment you stop pushing and taking chances where success is not guaranteed is the moment when you stop growing. Henry Ford said, *"whether or not you think you or can't do something, you are right!"* It really is about what you believe, good or bad. Once you get over your initial fear everything gets easier afterwards.

Surround Yourself with Positive People

"You are the average of the 5 people you spend the most time around." -Jim Rohn

Your thoughts and behavior are most influenced by your environment, the music, the television, radio, but most the people you spent time with. The people you spend time with whether they are co-workers, family, friends, etc. are the people you share and exchange ideas with. They often reinforce your thoughts because people tend to spend time with those they have the most in common. When Jim Rohn said, *"You are the average of the 5 people you spend the most time around,"* it makes perfect sense because people of a like mind and culture congregate. If you want a wealth mindset and more income, spend *less* time with people who don't have one and *more* time with those that do. Even if it's family and friends, you must spend more time with other people who are on the same journey as you. Otherwise, you will have the same income, same life and same experience as they do.

Change Your Inputs

If you are spending *less* time with people who *don't* share your common goals, you must replace that time with new information, new thoughts, new ideas. Go to the library get books. If you are not a reader, get audio cd's. Listen to podcasts, use your commute to and from work as your "auto university" instead of the radio. Spend more time at the bookstore. Make a treat of it. Get excited about learning some new to make you and your family wealthier.

Celebrate Your Successes

> "Where there is joy, there is success."
> **-Alex B Jones**

A lot of people have the wrong idea about success and winning. People mistakenly think in order to be successful you can't have fun. It simply isn't true. Yes, success requires a certain level of consistency, commitment, and discipline. But success is also about joy, having fun. Have you ever played a game and suddenly found yourself losing? When you lose more than you win, are you having fun? Usually not.

That's what happens to many beauty professionals in business and life. If over time you are not winning (succeeding) in your business, it becomes less fun. Pretty soon you have no joy and you're no longer passionate about what you have been gifted to do. It's hard to make other people feel great when you feel crummy on the inside. The cure is to get committed, exercise some discipline and consistency and be prepared to be amazed at how great it feels to win.

KEYS TO SUCCESS

1. Face your fears. Believe in yourself, think positively and be grateful for all that is coming to you
2. Be intentional in your thoughts and actions
3. Learn as much as you can about money. Look for and engage in activities that increase your income
4. Never feel guilty for charging for your services and know you are worthy of riches and abundance
5. Connect with people who are on the same path as you.
6. Invest in yourself and your future
7. Never think in lack only abundance. Don't fit your life into a small budget. Build big income for a big life.
8. Inform one person who is depending on you <u>and</u> one person who can advise you on reaching your stated goal.

STEP 2
"6-FIGURE MATH" & SET YOUR TARGETS

"By the inch, it's a cinch. By the mile, it takes a while."
-Anon

Perhaps the main reason why most people aren't more successful is they don't take the time to set goals for themselves and determine how it might be possible for them to achieve it. Most hairstylists bounce around aimlessly just getting by living paycheck to paycheck. Without vision people perish. You see, it is next to impossible to hit a target you can't see or a goal you haven't set. Once you set a target, the universe will begin to work on achieving these goals. You'll be amazed at how easy increasing your income becomes when you set a target and break it down.

Now that you are thinking more positively and being more intentional about your income, now we can begin setting goals to direct your focus, resources, time and efforts.

What is success?

> **suc·cess** - (n) the achievement of or progress towards something desired, planned, or attempted.

It is literally impossible to have success without a target or goal. Goals give us direction. Say for instance you were going on a trip. The destination becomes the goal. If you've never been to that place before, the first thing you would probably do is look up exactly where it is. You'd pull out a map, google or put it in your phone's GPS to determine where it is and how you plan to get there.

It works the same way in business. You must first determine what your goal is. Once you've determined what is important for you to achieve, then you can set goals and then develop your plan or strategy to get there. If it's important enough for you to map out your trip to go across town, isn't it important enough to do the same for success in our business?

Use the following pages to do your "6-Figure" math and set your income targets. Even if you are far from your goal now, you'll see by going through this exercise, how you can and will reach this goal. You're probably closer to the goal of making 6 figures than you realize. But you have to do the math.

Let's break it down.

6-Figure Math

Example:

Yearly Income You Desire $100,000

Workdays a week 3

Hours per workday 10

How many weeks of vacation? 3

52 weeks – 3 weeks = 49 work weeks per year

How much must you earn per week?

$100,000 / 49 weeks = $2,040/week

How much must you earn per day?

$2,040 a week / 3 workdays a week = $680/day

How much must you earn per hour?

$680 a day / 10 hours a day = $68/hour

Here are your weekly, daily, and hourly targets?

Weekly	$2,040
Daily	$680
Hour	$68

Weekly Income Target $2,040/week

**What is the average amount you currently
receive per client?** $68/client
(the total amount you currently make per week divided by the number of clients service for the week)

You must service this many clients per week   30 per week

How many clients do you need in your client base?

Clients per week	How often clients visit	Total clients needed
30	every 2 weeks	60
30	every 3 weeks	90
30	every 4 weeks	120
30	every 5 weeks	150
30	every 6 weeks	180

How large of a clientele must you have to achieve your income goals? _____

(Our goal for this book of $100,000 a year working 3 days per week)

Now that you've done the "6-Figure Math", aren't you amazed at just how simple earning at least a $100k a year actually is? By purchasing this book and doing the "6-Figure" math, you are much closer than 81% of the people in the Beauty Industry who never set their intention and purpose on making more money and accumulating wealth.

Yearly Income You Desire $_____ (A)

Workdays per week   _____ days

Hours per workday   _____ hours

How many weeks of vacation?

    52 weeks − _____ weeks of vacation = _____ (B) work wks/yr

How much must you earn per week?

    $__(A)____ / _(B)___ weeks = $_____ /week

How much must you earn per day?

    $____ a week / __ workdays a week = $___/day

How much must you earn per hour?

    $___ a day / __ hours a day = $__/hour

Here are your weekly, daily, and hourly targets?

    Weekly $_____
    Daily $_____
    Hour $_____

Yearly Income You Desire $_____ (A)

Workdays per week   _____ days

Hours per workday   _____ hours

How many weeks of vacation?

  52 weeks − _____ weeks of vacation = _____ (B) work wks/yr

How much must you earn per week?

  $ __(A)__ / __(B)__ weeks = $_____ /week

How much must you earn per day?

  $____ a week / __ workdays a week = $___/day

How much must you earn per hour?

  $___ a day / __ hours a day = $__/hour

Here are your weekly, daily, and hourly targets?

  Weekly $_____
  Daily $_____
  Hour $_____

Yearly Income You Desire $_____ (A)

Workdays per week   _____ days

Hours per workday   _____ hours

How many weeks of vacation?

52 weeks − _____ weeks of vacation = _____(B) work wks/yr

How much must you earn per week?

$__(A)____ / __(B)___ weeks = $_____ /week

How much must you earn per day?

$____ a week / __ workdays a week = $____/day

How much must you earn per hour?

$___ a day / __ hours a day = $__/hour

Here are your weekly, daily, and hourly targets?

Weekly	$_____
Daily	$_____
Hour	$_____

Weekly Income Target $____/week

**What is the average amount you
currently receive per client?** $__/client

(the total amount you currently make per week divided by the number of clients serviced for the week)

**You must service this
number of clients per week** __ per week

How many clients do you need total in your client base?

Clients per week	How often clients visit	Total clients needed
_____	_____	_____
_____	_____	_____
_____	_____	_____
_____	_____	_____
_____	_____	_____

How large of a clientele must you have to achieve your income goals? _____

(Our goal for this book of $100,000 a year working 3 days per week

Weekly Income Target $____/week

**What is the average amount you
currently receive per client?** $___/client

(the total amount you currently make per week divided by the number of clients serviced for the week)

**You must service this
number of clients per week**   ___ per week

How many clients do you need total in your client base?

Clients per week	How often clients visit	Total clients needed
_____	_____	_____
_____	_____	_____
_____	_____	_____
_____	_____	_____
_____	_____	_____

How large of a clientele must you have to achieve your income goals? _____

(Our goal for this book of $100,000 a year working 3 days per week)

Weekly Income Target $_____/week

What is the average amount you currently receive per client? $___/client

(the total amount you currently make per week divided by the number of clients serviced for the week)

You must service this number of clients per week ___ per week

How many clients do you need total in your client base?

Clients per week	How often clients visit	Total clients needed
_____	_____	_____
_____	_____	_____
_____	_____	_____
_____	_____	_____
_____	_____	_____

How large of a clientele must you have to achieve your income goals? _____

(Our goal for this book of $100,000 a year working 3 days per week)

Now that you have the "6-figure math" done for your salon business and you have it broken into down into your quarterly, monthly, weekly and daily targets, you can determine the top 3 things you should do daily and weekly basis so you never lose focus or get overwhelmed on your journey to greater success.

Commitment Determines Your Destiny

How committed are you to making more money and your success? The truth is whether or not you reach the level of success you want is directly related to your level of commitment. Success requires consistency. Many of lose focus, interest or become overwhelmed in the process of attaining their goals. Can you stay focused? Can you remain committed to the process even when you don't feel like it? Your level of commitment will determine your destiny.

On the next page is The 6-Figure Statement of Commitment. Complete and sign your Statement of Commitment only when you are truly committed to the process of achieving your goals.

STATEMENT OF COMMITMENT

I will maximize my full potential and become a _____ earning beauty professional. I will earn $_____ by providing exceptional value to my ideal clients working _____ days a week.

I am completely confident I can and will accomplish this goal by _____(date). I commit to doing at least

_____,

_____,

_____

to reach my goals. I will be successful in reaching my goal.

Signed _____

Date _____

KEYS TO SUCCESS

1. Write your 3 most important goals down in clear details and when you will achieve them
2. Do the "6-Figure" Math. See your big income goals in small manageable targets.
3. Set your yearly, weekly and daily income targets
4. Set the date you will achieve your income goals and working backwards determine what needs to be done
5. Fully commit to achieving by consistently performing all the activities outlined
6. Keep your goals with you at all times
7. Identify the activities you should concentrate on to give you the highest and best results towards your goals.
8. Track your daily and weekly results and celebrate your progress

STEP 3
WHAT'S YOUR STORY?

"There's no greater agony than bearing an untold story inside you."
-Maya Angelou

The Beauty Industry has become extremely competitive over the last few years and the number of people joining the ranks and pace of competition is expected to increase over the next decade. To remain competitive as a beauty professional and create more success for yourself, you will need more than great hairstyling ability to thrive in this cut-throat business environment. The marketplace needs to who you are, what you do and have a clear idea of how what you do will benefit them. In essence, "what's your story?"

What is "Your Story"?

The biggest challenge most beauty professionals must overcome is their lack of marketing and sells skills. Ask many hairstylist and they'll most likely tell you they didn't sign up for this career to be some sleazy, pushy salesperson. But, if you're like most beauty professionals, you probably also need to attract more clients to your salon business. Without a keen understanding of marketing and selling, you and your salon business will likely suffer.
To attract the right people to your business, there must be a signal or message that goes out to grab their attention and compel them to listen to you. A company's story is critical to their

success. In fact, you can't have a powerful brand without "the story."

"Your story" gives the authentic message of

- who you are,
- what you do or provide,
- who you do it for,
- why you are driven to do what you do,
- your culture,
- your values,
- what people can expect to receive from you and
- the manner they will receive it.

This is actually what is part of Marketing more specifically "positioning" your brand. Without a well-crafted story, it will be difficult to attract more of the right people to your service and brand. Think about Apple, Harley Davidson, Paul Mitchell or Olaplex. Each of these companies spend a lot of time thinking, crafting "their story." about their messaging - who they are, what they do, what do we want to be known for, their style, etc.

Not only is developing a clear "story" of who you are necessary to attract clients, it also helpful to you and other people who might be instrumental in helping you achieve your business goals. To generate more money, you must be consistent. "Your story" reminds you of who you are when you aren't feeling like yourself. Tell your story to everyone, including yourself, over and over, the same way every time.

In this step, you will develop your Marketing Message and Tagline to attract your ideal clients. This will help you be consistent in your messaging, help establish your brand in the marketplace and give you confidence when you are communicating with potential clients.

The first step in attracting more clients to your business, starts with gaining the attention of those you want to do business with. Once you've gained their attention, you must have something compelling to say and something that resonates with them. So they will continue to listen.

What do you do?
_____
_____
_____

Who do you help?
_____
_____
_____

What are their BIGGEST problems, issues or challenges?
_____
_____
_____

What do you or your company "stand against"?
_____
_____

What is your or your salon's "purpose"?
_____
_____
_____

Why should they do business with you?
_____
_____
_____

How do you SOLVE those issues or relieve their pain?
_____
_____

What service(s) do you prefer performing the most? (In order)
1.
2.
3.
So, here the marketing message formula.

I'm a _____ (your title)

I help _____ (your ideal client)

(do or have what) _____

so they can (do what) _____.

Here's mine...

> *"I'm a licensed cosmetologist. I help busy, professional women who want their own hair to be beautiful, healthy and easy to maintain with timely and exceptional salon experiences so they can look and feel more beautiful."*

As you can see, I'm pretty clear on who I'm looking for and who my ideal client is. As I share my message, professional women who are busy, don't have time to waste in a salon, who don't wear weaves or extensions know they can count on me to give them timely and exceptional salon experiences. And they know their hair will be beautiful, healthy and easy to maintain.

How do they know? Because I just told them. Deliver on your market message and you'll be successful.

Tagline

People have very short attention spans. They're evaluating from the moment they meet you if you are worthy of their time. You have to give them something worth paying attention pretty quick or they're gone. That's where taglines come in. A tagline is a short intriguing statement that makes them want to engage with you more. Also, if you have limited amount of space and you are trying to communicate your message, taglines work great. A tagline really is like a shorten version of your marketing message.

Here's my tagline:

"I make women look and feel beautiful."

After telling people this, they always ask, really? How?

And then I give them the marketing message.

> *"I'm a licensed cosmetologist. I help busy, professional women who want their own hair to be beautiful healthy and easy to maintain with timely and exceptional salon experiences so they can look and feel more beautiful."*

Write out your marketing message and tagline.

_____
_____
_____
_____
_____
_____
_____
_____

KEYS TO SUCCESS

1. Understand attracting and retaining clients is your #1 job in your business
2. Identify what you do best and what you want your business to be known for
3. Identify exactly who you want to do business with and what's important to them.
4. Develop a compelling, authentic story about who you are, what you do and how your service can change their world
5. Become very familiar with your marketing message. Commit it to memory.
6. Educate or give potential clients something of value before trying to recruit them
7. Share your message and use it everywhere and often with enthusiasm and confidence
8. Have fun and celebrate your accomplishments

STEP 4
MAXIMIZING CLIENT VALUE

"Know what your customers want most and what you do best.
Focus on where those two meet."
-Kevin Stirtz

You may not realize it but you have actually accomplished a lot in very short period of time. You are adapting a high-earning, 6-figure mindset to attract income to you through intentional thoughts, beliefs and money habits. You have identified who your target market is and created a powerful, compelling marketing message. Now, it's time to make things happen.

People mistakenly think earning a 6-figure income must be complicated and difficult. When you get down to it, there are really only a few different ways to grow your salon business. For this book, we will concentrate on the most important and foundational strategies to significantly increasing your income and creating freedom in your salon business....*fast*!

Use one or any combination of the following strategies to reach your 6-Figure goals to create all the income and freedom you want. I recommend implementing these strategies in this order to get fastest results and experience the least about of disruption to your clients.

One of the fastest and most effective ways to generate more income in your salon business is to leverage what you currently have and maximize the value you deliver to your current clients. You will do this by a concept I call "Up-Servicing". Up-Servicing is similar to up-selling except it is *only* focused on delivering greater value to the client and only recommending services and products that in the client's best interest and not that of the salon.

This is an important distinction. See, I know when it comes to recommending additional services and products to their clients, many hairstylists feel like they're being pushy or sleazy. But let me ask you, have you ever had someone over hear a conversation about additional services and products and they ask, "why didn't you recommend that for me?"

You see your clients want what's best for them. They want the latest and greatest. They want the things that are going to going to make them look and feel their best. By *not* offering additional services and products, you're not doing your clients a favor. You're actually doing them a disservice. Their hair color doesn't last as long, it isn't as shiny or it's limp and has no volume. Clients want to know about the latest and greatest to help them look their best. In addition, it's not the best representation of your work. You can hardly expect many referrals or to grow your business that way. You see it only when you are not recommending services and products in their best interest that's when the sleazy begins to creep in.

Your goal is to recommend 1 additional service and/or 1 additional product with each client visit. Remember, your average service ticket amount per client needs to be a minimum $68 if you work 3 days and service 30 clients a week.

Consider putting together service and retail bundles. That's a great way to add value to the client and increase your revenue.

Here's how to recommend additional services and products without feeling sleazy or pushy.

Use this script.
(Call at the beginning of the week Sunday or Monday when you preparing for your week)

> **Hey _____ how are you?**
>
> ***I'm looking forward to seeing you on _____ at _____ time.***
>
> ***I'm calling because you're very important to me and I want to make sure I'm giving you the absolute best service.***

I was looking over your last few visits and I noticed we (haven't done a/you haven't had a...service) _____.

I recommend we schedule a _____.

It's only $_____ it takes x minutes and you'll love the _____ (benefit)

Awesome!
I look forward to seeing you!

To help your client maintain their look, here are the products she/he will need:

_____

_____

After your client's service, ask how he/she likes it. Always respond positively. Now that you're sure he/she likes their hair, recommend the 2 products she needs to maintain her look, shine, resist fading, etc.
Here's how...

_____, how do you like your hair/style/cut/color?

What do you like most about it?

Me too. In order to maintain _____ (whatever she said she liked most), I

recommend _____ & _____

to _____ (do what).

Do you any questions about how or how much to use?

Awesome!

Practice these scripts. Remember, if you are not recommending products and services you're doing your clients a disservice.

KEYS TO SUCCESS

1. Up-service not up-sell. Only recommend products and services in the best interest of your clients
2. You are doing your clients a disservice by NOT recommending additional services and products
3. Clients you recommend services and products to are happier with their salon experience
4. Recommend services to your clients ahead of time so they can be prepared to purchase
5. Recommend products after you're sure clients are happy with their look and experience
6. Make at least 1 product or service recommendation to <u>every</u> client, <u>every</u> visit
7. Remember "NO" just means "not now". Simply ask again at their next visit.
8. Celebrate yourself every time you ask

STEP 5
INCREASING YOUR FOV's

"Customer satisfaction is worthless. Customer loyalty is priceless."
-Jeffery Gitomer

Increasing the frequency of your clients' salon visits (FOV) is the next best way to help them always look and feel their absolute best. It also means less work, and more income for you as well. Clients usually defer to your recommendations when it comes to scheduling salon visits. If you find clients are a reluctant to your recommendations, it may be time to reestablish yourself as the expert. Educate and share information with your clients about new styles, services and products. Send a newsletter or share articles that would interest them and reestablish yourself as a knowledgeable and credible resource.

Increasing your clients from a 5-week to a 4-week schedule means they will go from coming 10 times a year to 13. If on average each client spends $100 per visit, then you've just earned an extra $300 for the year. Move 10 clients up by 1 week and you just added $3,000 for the year. Awesome!

Here's how you do it. At the end of their service after you've shared with them your product recommendations, *pick a week* sooner than they normally come and say.

Let's schedule you for _____ (day/week)

Same time? _____

Or, I noticed you normally come every x weeks and your _____(color/cut/etc.) doesn't get _____ (some benefit) and I want to make sure you _____ (another benefit). Let's schedule same day and time on _____date.

Awesome!

See you then.

Another approach to increasing the frequency of your clients' visits is by developing loyalty promotions. Offering a discount on salon services and even products when clients come back more often or purchase more products within a specified period of time increases your income. For example, if you produce a loyalty card with 10 visits before a certain date, they'll receive 15% off each visit *or* even the last one free. It's important to do the math to determine exactly how the promotion will work well for you and your guests.

KEYS TO SUCCESS

1. Look at how often each client visits your salon
2. Calculate how many times will they visit in a year
3. Calculate how many times a year would they visit if you moved them up just one week
4. Like a doctor, tell them when you want to see them again don't leave it up to them
5. Clearly communicate the benefits of moving them up one week.
6. Prepare an email or simple text message that you can send ahead of their next visit to get clients coming in sooner
7. Consider creating a VIP class or category of clients as an acknowledgement and reward for frequent guests.
8. **As always, celebrate every ask**

STEP 6
BUILDING YOUR CLIENTELE

"Help enough other people get what they want, you'll have everything you want in life."

-Zig Ziglar

You have determined you need to attract more clients. Using the formulas in step 2, you now know exactly how many you need to reach your income goals.

In step 3, you identified exactly who you want to business with and why they should do business with you. Using your new marketing message and tagline, you are now ready to start attracting your ideal clients.

Here are the next steps to follow:

1. Put your marketing message and/or tagline on everything; business cards, website, voicemail, email signature line, everywhere you use your name and brand

2. Commit your marketing message to memory and practice it.

3. Go through your phone, email contacts, online and social media contacts, groups organizations you are a member of. Using the next few pages make a list of all the people you would like to contact.

4. Put your contacts in different lists, those you know very well, people you know but haven't talk with in a while, and people you don't know but should.

5. Call old clients you want to reconnect with and haven't seen in a while.

6. Contact at least 3-5 people per day online and offline. Ask each person for a referral.

Here's how to get more referrals from your current clients:

> *By the way _____(VIP client). I love having you as my client. I'd like to do something special for you.*
>
> *I like to give one of your friends, family members or coworkers a _____(a gift card) compliments of you?*
>
> *Who would you like to receive it?*
>
> *Awesome!*
>
> *What's her name and phone number?*

When contacting the referred person. Here's what you say...

> *Hi! May I speak to _____. My name is _____ owner of _____ Salon. I was calling to let you your (friend/family/member/coworker) _____ is a client of mine and she has given you a gift card to our salon.*
>
> *What day would you like to receive your gift?*

Bonus Tip: Never ask "If" they know of somebody who wants (blah, blah).

This is a terrible way to ask for a referral. Here's a script I've been using that has always worked well and helped hundreds of hairstylists get more referrals. Commit this to memory.

> **WHO do you know, a friend, neighbor, someone you work with,** *(give ideas here to jog their thinking)* **, who maybe not now but sometime in the future want beautiful, healthy hair that's easy to maintain?**

This works well for several reasons:

- You asked "WHO" not "IF". "IF" gives them an easy way to say no they don't. "Who" is a direct ask for a person.
- You gave ideas of people who might be a good fit
- You said who want something not right now but in the future
- Finally, you inserted your marketing message again reinforcing what you do and who you're looking for. When you state it this way, who doesn't want beautiful hair.

Works like a charm, if you commit it to memory and use it often.

Top 7 Ways to Attract New Customers

Having a system for attracting more clients to your business is extremely important to the overall success of your business.

1. **Referrals.** Developing a strong referral system is best way to build a solid, steady clientele. As a marketing strategy getting referrals is 5 times cheaper, referred clients spend more and they remain a client longer.

2. **Reactivating Old/Lost Clients.** Reconnecting and reactivating your long lost clients can also be a great way to build your clientele. Clients may have been thinking about you but had not reached out just yet. Calling, texting or emailing to check in and reconnect with them and say hello can be the beginning of reactivated relationship.

3. **Facebook Ads and Boosted Posts.** Ads and boosted posts are a great and inexpensive way to attract new clients to your salon. You can be very targeted with who sees your ads and how much money you spend. Run your ad as long as you want. Check in mind the objective of your ad and build your copy and creative piece to match the outcome you want.

4. **Video Marketing.** Marketing yourself and your business with video content is the next best thing to people talking to you in person. Video is a powerfully medium to share who you are, what you do, and the benefits your clients receive. You highlight your expertise and even educate potential clients.

5. **Email Marketing.** Use email in conjunction with facebook ads and video marketing to build up your list of people who want to connect and engage with you. It is important that you build your email list as a marketing approach so you don't have to

continue to pay to advertise to them on Facebook, Instagram or other social media platforms.

6. **Open House/Seminars**. Hosting seminars, open house and other events is a great way for clients to bring people who bring potential referrals to and is a nice easy way for them to meet you without feeling obligated.

7. **Partnerships**. If you need more clients, one of the best ways to attract more is to partner with another company or service provider who has a client base similar to the people you service. Working a partner to build up each other's portfolio is a powerful and effective way to get the clients you want for your business.

If you would like more information on how to attract more clients to your salon business easily and automatically with little to no money, go to www.alexbjones.com/6figurebookresources.

KEYS TO SUCCESS

1. Understand that building your clientele is no one responsibility but yours
2. Make a clientele-building activities a top priority in your salon business daily
3. Look at how many people you need to attract to your business
4. Commit these scripts to memory
5. Practice with your family, friends, colleagues to get better with asking for referrals
6. Make a habit of talking to 3 to 5 people a day and ask for a referral
7. When asking for a referral, always ask "who do you know" rather than "if you know someone"
8. Remember, if you don't ask you won't receive

STEP 7
"ADJUSTING" YOUR PRICES

Now we've come to what beauty professionals fear the most...the dreaded *price increases.* Know and understand that you can't run successful business off your passion for what you do and love for your clients. Love on them and give them the absolute best service. Then charge them accordingly! Too many of us think, I'll be able to attract and do more people if my prices are low. Repeat after me, YOU CAN'T WORK YOUR WAY OUT OF BAD PRICING! If your operating expenses are not low as well, you will only cut your own throat and stunt the growth of your business. This is probably the second biggest reason hairstylist go out of business, not charging appropriately.

If you don't charge correctly, you
- will work harder and longer than you have to
- will attract the wrong clients...(cheap ones)
- won't have the resources to provide high end services
- can't afford to get education to build your business
- will not have enough revenue to sustain, and grow your business
- you and your family will suffer unnecessarily.

Profit is not a bad word. In business, it is critical to your survival and the survival of your business.

Reasons Why Most Hairstylists Are Afraid to Adjust Their Prices

- Fear of losing clients
- Negative reactions from clients
- Don't have a system for replacing lost clients and attracting new customers
- Guilt and worry
- Don't know what to charge
- Don't know what to say to adjust their prices
- Feeling of unworthiness

All of these fears and feelings all stem from not knowing how and when to adjust your prices and how to market your business. You see, if you have a whole list of clients who are trying to get in with you and pay top dollar, it would be highly unlikely that you be as concerned about a few clients grumbling over your prices going up and threatening to leave. You wouldn't care as much. But when you feel like you already don't have enough, you feel the most important thing to do is hang on to the clients you have rather than raise your prices and risk losing them.

This is a lack mentality! There are thousands of other people out there many who want to be their service provider and willing to pay you more money. Overcome this fear by building a pipeline of people who want to do business with you.

Are any of the following conditions true:

- are you at least 80% booked
- has it been more than 12 months since you adjusted your prices
- have you had a significant increase in operating expenses
- you've added any new upgrades to your salon, services or amenities
- you can't reach your weekly income goal working the number of days you want at your current average service ticket amount

It's time to adjust your salon prices.

Here's where so many of us get stuck. How much? When? Who to charge? On what services? Once these questions start swirling around in their heads, most stylists just settle for asking their colleagues what they charge. Once this happens, it starts the downward spiral into settling into being average and mediocre. You'll get what everyone else gets when you charge what other people.

Do not fall into that trap! Make your income expand to the lifestyle you want instead of fitting your life into a small budget. So, without making this too complicated, let's go back to our "6-Figure" Math in Chapter 2.

6-Figure Math

Yearly Income You Desire $100,000

Workdays a week 3

Hours per workday 10

How many weeks of vacation? 3

    52 weeks – 3 weeks = 49 work weeks per year

How much must you earn per week?

    $100,000 / 49 weeks = $2,040/week

How much must you earn per day?

    $2,040 a week / 3 workdays a week = $680/day

How much must you earn per hour?

    $680 a day / 10 hours a day = $68/hour

Here are your weekly, daily, and hourly targets?

Weekly	$2,040
Daily	$680
Hour	$68 ⬅

In this example, we need to make a minimum of $68 an hour to reach our income goal. So, this is amount we should be charging for our services. Of course, you are going to do the 6-Figure Math for your salon business and determine what you should be charging for your services.

Service	Minimum Price
15 min services	$17
30 min services	$34
1-hour services	$68
1 ½ hour services	$102
2-hour services	$136

*Add in product costs for color, special conditioners, hair, extensions, etc.

These are minimum prices for salon services based on service time and income goals. Think about how and where you can increase the value of the services you deliver to your clients. If you choose to charge more, even better. If you work with only 1 client at a time working 3 days a week, 10 hours per day, you will earn $100,000 for the year.

KEYS TO SUCCESS

1. This is your business. You must charge a price high enough to meet your business and personal financial goals
2. Never ask what other hairstylists are charging. They don't have a reason or strategy for their pricing
3. Understand that pricing communicates how you feel about yourself. You deserve to be wealthy
4. Understand that pricing communicates how you feel about yourself and the service you provide
5. Price is what your client pays for the service. Value is what they actually receive.
6. You can't work your way out of bad pricing
7. If you don't charge appropriately you'll never achieve freedom in your salon business
8. Give yourself permission to succeed

STEP 8
TRACKING YOUR PROGRESS

"Wealth is the result of vision, intention, and effort done well repeatedly and consistently."

You've come to the final step in creating a 6-figure income for yourself: tracking your progress. This may seem like a boring and unnecessary step. But, this process is so important to your overall success.

As with any game, the only way you know if you're winning is to keep score. If you don't keep score, you don't know if you are ahead or behind, gaining or losing ground. Tracking your progress allows you to see if you are being consistent, what activities you are doing, what results you're getting and it helps you see what's working and what you need to change to get greater results.

How to Use The 6-Figure Salonpreneur™ Progress Tracker

On the next page, you'll notice that the Progress Tracker is designed for the week. It is sized so you can keep it with you on your 6-Figure journey. Think of it as your map or GPS system. You wouldn't look at your map or GPS and then leave it at home would you? With The Tracker, you're able to plan out your week and schedule the activities most important to reaching your 6-Figure income goals. It's also flexible enough for you to add those items and activities you think are important in addition to the ones provided.

Do you ever feel like you're confused, overwhelmed or just don't get as much done as you would like? Without a doubt, its because you haven't carved out what needs to be done and when. If ever the results you're getting aren't as intended, the first place you should is at your 6-Figure Salonpreneur™ Progress Tracker. Did you follow through on what you needed to consistently? Did you make any changes or tweaks? What working and what's not? Your 6-Figure Salonpreneur™ Progress Tracker will be your first indicator of success.

1. Start at the beginning of the week, preferably Sunday and look at what you have scheduled and compare that to your income goals.
2. Use any combination of the 4 steps outlined in this book to increase your income for the week.
3. Send out emails, newsletters, etc. to build your work schedule for the week
4. Call clients on your off days to recommend additional services.
5. Schedule when and how you're going to meet new people
6. Write all your activities throughout the day
7. Create a legend at the bottom of The 6-Figure Tracker and note them in the worksheet in the proper space

8. Do the most important and most difficult items on your daily planner first.
9. Get in the habit of doing your totals at the end of each day
10. Celebrate
11. Make adjustments as needed the next day to reach your income goals.

You have been given everything you need to generate the income and have the life you want. Use this information to get the income, freedom and life you deserve. It's up to you! I look forward to seeing you at the top!

Be great!
Alex

THE 6- FIGURE SALONPRENEUR™
TRACKING YOUR PROGRESS

	S	M	T	W	TH	F	S	Totals
Daily $ Goal				$680	$680	$680		$2,040
Daily Activities								
1		Call client	Network	Call new	1 product	FOV		
2				upservice				
3	newsletter			rebook				
Social Media	Fb groups	FB 3 / IG 2	P2 FB 3 IG 1		Fb3 tw2			
New/Old Contacts		5new/2old	4new/3old					
New Clients				1	0	1		2
Service Total				$400	$498	$597		$1,495
Retail Sales Total				$92	$107	$110		$309
Daily Totals				$492	$605	$707		$1,804
+/-				-$188	-$75	+$27		-$236

KEYS TO SUCCESS

1. Start on your day off at the beginning of the week.

2. Assess what actions went well last week and what needs to change for the coming week

3. Always keep with this book with you to review your goals, scripts, take notes and track results

4. Input your numbers throughout each day.

5. Always close out each day daily and at the end of each week

6. Make each goal something that can be easily measure like how many new people did you share the opportunity with to do business with you each day.

7. Record your numbers accurately. Don't fudge your numbers. It will be more beneficial to have accurate than numbers that look good

8. Review your progress with your accountability partner each week

ABOUT THE AUTHOR

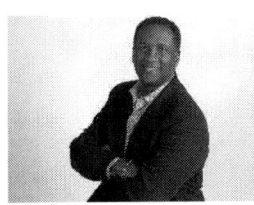 Alex Jones is Founder of The Salonpreneur™ Academy and Salon Business Coach specializing in helping independent hairstylists, booth renters, salon owners and salon suite owners get more clients, more income and more freedom in the salon business. Over the past 23 years, Alex has owned and operated 3 salons, worked as a platform artist and helped hundreds of beauty professional across the country finally live their dream. He is a speaker and marketing expert.

Prior to working in the Beauty Industry, Alex worked with Kodak Company as a Corporate Auditor and in Marketing and Product Development. He attended undergraduate and graduate school at Florida A&M University studying Economics and Finance. He lives in Rock Hill, South Carolina just outside of Charlotte, North Carolina.

ADDITIONAL TRAINING AND PRODUCTS

My goal is to help as many beauty professionals as possible attract more clients, generate more income and create the freedom you truly want in your business and your life. If you are tired and frustrated with the results you are getting in your salon business, I have additional training, products and coaching services available to help you finally have the business of your dreams.

Go to **www.alexbjones.com/6figurebookresources** and elevate your business today.

Salon Business Monthly Membership
Salon SuccessLab Monthly Membership

Online Products
Thrive Blueprint
Client Attraction Program
BREAKTHROUGH 28-Day Marketing Plan

Coaching
Elevate Program 6-Week Live Online Program
Power Hour 1-on-1 Coaching
Perfect Pricing Session

"Done-For-You" Services
Facebook Advertising
Salon Business Audit

Free Resources
6-Figure Salonpreneur™ Tracking Your Progress Worksheets

THE 6- FIGURE SALONPRENEUR™
TRACKING YOUR PROGRESS

WEEK _____

	S	M	T	W	TH	F	S	Total
Daily $ Goal								
Daily Activities								
1								
2								
3								
Social Media								
New/Old Contacts								
New Clients								
Service Total								
Retail Sales Total								
Daily Totals								
+/-								

THE 6- FIGURE SALONPRENEUR™
TRACKING YOUR PROGRESS

WEEK _____

	S	M	T	W	TH	F	S	Total
Daily $ Goal								
Daily Activities								
1								
2								
3								
Social Media								
New/Old Contacts								
New Clients								
Service Total								
Retail Sales Total								
Daily Totals								
+/-								

THE 6- FIGURE SALONPRENEUR™
TRACKING YOUR PROGRESS

WEEK _____

	S	M	T	W	TH	F	S	Total
Daily $ Goal								
Daily Activities								
1								
2								
3								
Social Media								
New/Old Contacts								
New Clients								
Service Total								
Retail Sales Total								
Daily Totals								
+/-								

THE 6- FIGURE SALONPRENEUR™
TRACKING YOUR PROGRESS
WEEK _____

	S	M	T	W	TH	F	S	Total
Daily $ Goal								
Daily Activities								
1								
2								
3								
Social Media								
New/Old Contacts								
New Clients								
Service Total								
Retail Sales Total								
Daily Totals								
+/-								

THE 6-FIGURE SALONPRENEUR™
TRACKING YOUR PROGRESS

WEEK _____

	S	M	T	W	TH	F	S	Total
Daily $ Goal								
Daily Activities								
1								
2								
3								
Social Media								
New/Old Contacts								
New Clients								
Service Total								
Retail Sales Total								
Daily Totals								
+/-								

THE 6- FIGURE SALONPRENEUR™
TRACKING YOUR PROGRESS

WEEK _____

	S	M	T	W	TH	F	S	Total
Daily $ Goal								
Daily Activities								
1								
2								
3								
Social Media								
New/Old Contacts								
New Clients								
Service Total								
Retail Sales Total								
Daily Totals								
+/-								

THE 6-FIGURE SALONPRENEUR™
TRACKING YOUR PROGRESS
WEEK _____

	S	M	T	W	TH	F	S	Total
Daily $ Goal								
Daily Activities								
1								
2								
3								
Social Media								
New/Old Contacts								
New Clients								
Service Total								
Retail Sales Total								
Daily Totals								
+/-								

THE 6- FIGURE SALONPRENEUR™
TRACKING YOUR PROGRESS

WEEK _____

	S	M	T	W	TH	F	S	Total
Daily $ Goal								
Daily Activities								
1								
2								
3								
Social Media								
New/Old Contacts								
New Clients								
Service Total								
Retail Sales Total								
Daily Totals								
+/-								

THE 6-FIGURE SALONPRENEUR™
TRACKING YOUR PROGRESS

WEEK _____

	S	M	T	W	TH	F	S	Total
Daily $ Goal								
Daily Activities								
1								
2								
3								
Social Media								
New/Old Contacts								
New Clients								
Service Total								
Retail Sales Total								
Daily Totals								
+/-								

THE 6- FIGURE SALONPRENEUR™
TRACKING YOUR PROGRESS

WEEK _____

	S	M	T	W	TH	F	S	Total
Daily $ Goal								
Daily Activities								
1								
2								
3								
Social Media								
New/Old Contacts								
New Clients								
Service Total								
Retail Sales Total								
Daily Totals								
+/-								

THE 6- FIGURE SALONPRENEUR™
TRACKING YOUR PROGRESS
WEEK ____

	S	M	T	W	TH	F	S	Total
Daily $ Goal								
Daily Activities								
1								
2								
3								
Social Media								
New/Old Contacts								
New Clients								
Service Total								
Retail Sales Total								
Daily Totals								
+/-								

THE 6-FIGURE SALONPRENEUR™
TRACKING YOUR PROGRESS

WEEK _____

	S	M	T	W	TH	F	S	Total
Daily $ Goal								
Daily Activities								
1								
2								
3								
Social Media								
New/Old Contacts								
New Clients								
Service Total								
Retail Sales Total								
Daily Totals								
+/-								

Made in the USA
Middletown, DE
09 July 2017